The Gallstone-Friendly Diet for Women

The Complete Nutritional Guide with Delicious Recipes to Stay Radiant, Resilient, and Enjoy a Healthier Life

DR LANA BROWN, RN

Copyright Page

© 2024 by Dr. Lana Brown.

Table of Contents

INTRODUCTION

You may have heard a lot about gallstones, their associated pain, and treatment options, but do you know what size of gallstone is considered large? Some people develop numerous tiny gallstones, while others may have just one large stone. The gallbladder, a small pouch located under the liver, stores bile, a fluid produced by the liver that aids digestion. When there is an excess of cholesterol in the bile, it can lead to the formation of gallstones.

Gallstones typically vary in size, commonly between 5-10 mm in diameter, which usually doesn't pose serious risks. However, stones larger than this size can be dangerous. When gallstones block the bile ducts, your gallbladder may spasm, causing sharp, cutting pain. This intense pain can be so severe that it may feel like a heart attack, making it hard to catch your breath.

Gallstone pain may start shortly after eating, wake you from sleep, last from 15 minutes to several hours, and come and go over weeks, months, or even years. Once a gallbladder attack starts, there's nothing you can do to stop it, but the pain usually subsides if the stone moves through the bile duct on its own. If gallstones get stuck, they can cause severe spasms, increasing your heart rate and dropping your blood pressure, leading to dizziness. Prolonged blockage can cause inflammation or infection, making you feel extremely tired and sick.

While the exact cause of gallstones is unknown, they may form when:

There's too much cholesterol in your bile. Normally, bile dissolves cholesterol, but when it can't, the extra cholesterol builds up and forms stones.

There's too much bilirubin in your bile. Conditions like liver disease, infections, and blood disorders can cause the liver to produce excess bilirubin.

Your gallbladder doesn't empty completely, making your bile very concentrated.

You are more likely to develop gallstones if you:

- Have a family history of them.
- Are a woman or assigned female at birth.
- Are over 40.

- Are of Native American or Mexican descent.

- Have obesity.

- Consume a diet high in fat and cholesterol but low in fiber.

- Don't get much exercise.

- Use estrogen-based birth control or hormone replacement therapy.

- Take estrogen with feminizing hormone therapy.

- Have diabetes.

- Have an intestinal disease such as Crohn's.

- Have hemolytic anemia or cirrhosis of the liver.

- Take medication to lower cholesterol.

- Lose a significant amount of weight quickly, such as after weight loss surgery.

- Frequently fast.

CHAPTER I

UNDERSTANDING GALLSTONES

Gallstones, or cholelithiasis, are hardened deposits that form in the gallbladder or bile ducts, with a notably higher prevalence in women compared to men. The term "gallstone" combines "gall," meaning bile, and "stone," indicating the solid nature of these deposits. The gallbladder stores bile produced by the liver, which is then transported through bile ducts to aid in digestion. Gallstones form when components of bile, such as cholesterol or bilirubin, crystallize and clump together.

Globally, gallstones affect approximately 20% of adults, but the condition is significantly more common in women. In the United States, around 10% of adults have gallstones, with up to 75% of these individuals being women or people assigned female at birth (AFAB). This heightened prevalence in women is largely attributed to hormonal factors. For instance, estrogen, which fluctuates during pregnancy and with the use of hormonal contraceptives, can alter bile composition and gallbladder function, increasing the risk of gallstone formation.

Despite the high prevalence, many women with gallstones are asymptomatic. However, about 20% of those diagnosed will experience symptoms or require treatment. Gallstones can lead to acute pain, often referred to as a gallbladder attack or gallstone attack, especially after eating when the gallbladder contracts. This pain is frequently described as intense, sharp, and cramping, and can be severe enough to disrupt sleep. The condition is marked by episodic pain known as biliary colic, which can last from minutes to hours and may subside when the stone moves or pressure in the biliary tract decreases.

The growth of gallstones can exacerbate their potential to cause problems. What begins as a small grain of sand can gradually increase in size as bile continues to deposit additional layers of sediment. This growth can eventually obstruct bile flow, particularly if the stone becomes lodged in a narrow bile duct or the neck of the gallbladder, leading to significant pain and potential complications.

Understanding the impact of gallstones on women is essential for developing effective management strategies and raising awareness. Women's higher susceptibility to gallstones underscores the need for targeted prevention and treatment approaches to address this common and potentially debilitating condition.

Types of Gallstones

Gallstones, which are particularly prevalent among women, come in two main types: cholesterol stones and pigment stones. Cholesterol stones, which are often yellow-green, are predominantly composed of hardened cholesterol. In many regions, these make up about 75% of all gallstones. Women are especially prone to cholesterol stones due to hormonal fluctuations that affect bile composition.

Pigment stones, darker in color and made of bilirubin, are less common but can still affect women, sometimes appearing alongside cholesterol stones.

Causes and Risk Factors

Women face specific risk factors for developing gallstones, influenced by hormonal and physiological changes:

- Hormones: Women's hormonal changes during pregnancy, hormone replacement therapy, or the use of birth control pills can elevate estrogen levels. Increased estrogen can lead to higher cholesterol levels in bile and reduced gallbladder motility, raising the risk of gallstones.

- Obesity: Obesity is a significant risk factor for women. Excess body fat not only raises estrogen levels but also increases cholesterol in bile, contributing to gallstone formation.

- Age: Women are at greater risk during their fertile years, typically between ages 20 and 50. Although gallstones are more common in people over 60, women within this age range are particularly susceptible.

- Ethnicity: Native American women exhibit the highest rates of gallstones, likely due to genetic factors that increase cholesterol secretion in bile.

- Rapid Weight Loss: Women who undergo rapid weight loss, such as after bariatric surgery, face increased risk as the liver releases excess cholesterol into bile.

- Fasting: Extended fasting decreases gallbladder movement, concentrating bile with cholesterol. Women who frequently fast or follow restrictive diets may be at higher risk.

Additional factors like the use of cholesterol-lowering medications and diabetes, which can affect triglyceride levels, also contribute to the risk for women.

Symptoms and Diagnosis

Women with gallstones often experience symptoms that can be particularly distressing:

Gallbladder Attack: This sudden and severe pain, often occurring after meals, can be alarming. Women may experience nausea or vomiting along with intense, cramping pain, which might disrupt sleep.

Biliary Colic: Women may experience episodic pain that builds to a peak and then gradually fades. This pain can last from minutes to hours and is often described as sharp, cramping, or squeezing.

Diagnostic methods for Gallstones in women include:

Ultrasound: The primary imaging technique used to detect gallstones, revealing the presence of stones in the gallbladder.

Cholecystography: An X-ray procedure that shows how contrast fluid flows through the gallbladder.

Blood Tests: These tests check for signs of infection or complications related to gallstones.

CT Scan: Provides detailed images of the gallbladder and surrounding organs, useful for identifying complications.

ERCP: An endoscopic procedure using a dye to visualize bile ducts and identify blockages.

Sphincterotomy: This procedure helps stones pass into the intestine by widening the muscle sphincter.

When to Seek Medical Help

For women experiencing gallstone symptoms, timely medical attention is crucial:

Severe Abdominal Pain: If you experience intense pain in the upper right abdomen or shoulder, especially after eating, seek immediate medical help. This may indicate a gallbladder attack, which can be particularly distressing for women.

Persistent Symptoms: If you suspect recurrent pain or biliary colic, consult your healthcare provider. Women with these symptoms may require diagnostic tests to confirm gallstones and discuss treatment options.

Surgical intervention, such as gallbladder removal, is a common and effective treatment with a high success rate. Early diagnosis and treatment can help manage symptoms and prevent complications, offering relief and improving quality of life for women affected by gallstones.

CHAPTER II

SPECIAL CONSIDERATIONS FOR WOMEN TO PREVENT GALLSTONE

Gallstones are a significant health concern for women, with a large percentage of those affected being women due to their unique physiological and hormonal factors. Preventative measures are crucial to reduce the risk and manage the potential for gallstone formation.

Hormonal Influences on Gallstone Formation

Women's hormonal cycles, including menstruation, pregnancy, and menopause, significantly influence gallstone risk. Estrogen, which increases cholesterol in bile, and progesterone, which slows gallbladder emptying, both contribute to gallstone formation. This hormonal effect explains why women under 40 are diagnosed with gallstones almost three times more often than men. The risk decreases with age but remains higher for women due to the lingering effects of hormonal changes.

Dietary Adjustments During Menstruation, Pregnancy, and Menopause

Dietary Adjustments During Menstruation, Pregnancy, and Menopause

Diet plays a crucial role in managing and preventing gallstones, especially during hormonal shifts:

Menstruation: During menstruation, women might experience changes in bile composition due to hormonal fluctuations. Increasing fiber intake through fruits, vegetables, beans, and whole grains can help stabilize bile composition.

Pregnancy: Pregnancy increases the risk of gallstones due to elevated estrogen levels. Pregnant women should focus on a diet rich in healthy fats like fish oil and olive oil to help the gallbladder contract and empty regularly. Avoiding high-fat and fried foods is also beneficial.

Menopause: Hormonal replacement therapy (HRT) during menopause can increase gallstone risk. Women undergoing HRT should discuss dietary adjustments with their healthcare provider, focusing on high-fiber foods and healthy fats to mitigate risk.

Dietary choices play a crucial role in preventing gallstones in women. Experts recommend the following dietary adjustments to reduce the risk:

High-Fiber Foods: Incorporate more fruits, vegetables, beans, peas, and whole grains like brown rice, oats, and whole wheat bread.

Healthy Fats: Include healthy fats like fish oil and olive oil to promote regular gallbladder contraction and emptying.

Reduce Refined Carbohydrates and Sugar: Limit intake of refined carbs and sugary foods.

Avoid Unhealthy Fats: Cut down on unhealthy fats found in desserts and fried foods.

The Impact of Birth Control Pills and Hormone Replacement Therapy

Both birth control pills and hormone replacement therapy (HRT) can increase the risk of gallstones in women:

Birth Control Pills: Oral contraceptives slightly increase the risk of gallstones, particularly in the first decade of use. This is due to the increased levels of estrogen and progesterone, which can alter bile composition and gallbladder motility.

Hormone Replacement Therapy (HRT): HRT, especially when taken as a pill rather than a patch, significantly increases the risk of gallstones. Women on HRT should be vigilant about their diet and lifestyle to counteract this increased risk.

CHAPTER III

MANAGING GALLSTONE RISKS DURING PREGNANCY

Pregnancy significantly increases the risk of gallstones in women due to elevated levels of estrogen and progesterone. These hormones can increase cholesterol levels in bile and reduce gallbladder motility, leading to the formation of gallstones. It's crucial for pregnant women to be aware of this risk and take proactive steps to manage it.

Hormonal Impact:

- Estrogen: Increases cholesterol secretion, contributing to gallstone formation.

- Progesterone: Causes relaxation of muscle tissues, slowing bile release, which can lead to bile stasis and gallstone formation.

Symptoms to Watch For:

- Sharp pain in the upper abdomen after high-fat meals
- Pain between the shoulder blades or under the right shoulder
- Gas, abdominal bloating, sweating, chills, nausea, and vomiting

If you experience these symptoms, especially in the third trimester or postpartum, consult your healthcare provider. An ultrasound is the safest diagnostic tool for gallbladder issues during pregnancy.

Safe Dietary Practices for Pregnant Women

To manage and prevent gallstones during pregnancy, following safe dietary practices is essential:

Gain a Healthy Amount of Weight:

- Obesity is a significant risk factor for gallstones. Work with your healthcare provider to gain a healthy amount of weight during pregnancy.

Eat a High-Fiber Diet:

- Fiber-rich foods like fruits, vegetables, beans, and whole grains help maintain a healthy gallbladder. Aim to include these foods in your daily diet.

Choose Healthy Fats:

- Incorporate monounsaturated fats and omega-3 fats into your diet, found in foods like olive oil, fish, and nuts. These fats can help prevent gallstones.

Limit Sugar and Refined Carbohydrates:

- Reduce your intake of sugar and refined carbs like white bread, pasta, and sugary snacks, which can increase the risk of gallstones.

Manage Diabetes:

- If you have diabetes, work with your doctor to keep it under control. High triglyceride levels associated with diabetes can increase the risk of gallstones.

Postpartum Health and Gallstone Prevention

After delivering a baby, women may still be at increased risk of developing gallstones due to rapid weight loss and hormonal changes. To reduce this risk, it's important to continue following a healthy diet and lifestyle:

Maintain a Balanced Diet:

- Continue eating a high-fiber diet with healthy fats and low sugar to support gallbladder health.

Gradual Weight Loss:

- Avoid rapid weight loss after pregnancy. Aim for a gradual reduction in weight through a balanced diet and regular exercise.

Regular Physical Activity:

- Engage in moderate physical activity to help maintain a healthy weight and support overall health.

Monitor Symptoms:

- Be vigilant about any gallbladder-related symptoms and seek medical advice if they occur.

Menopause and Gallstones

Menopause brings significant hormonal changes that can increase the risk of gallstones. Estrogen levels decline, which can alter bile composition and gallbladder function. Here are some strategies to manage gallstone risks during menopause:

Monitor Hormone Replacement Therapy (HRT):

- HRT can increase the risk of gallstones. Discuss with your healthcare provider the risks and benefits of HRT, and explore alternative options if necessary.
- Healthy Diet:
- Continue following a diet rich in fiber, healthy fats, and low in sugar and refined carbs to support gallbladder health.

Regular Check-ups:

- Regular medical check-ups can help monitor gallbladder health and catch any issues early.

Lifestyle Adjustments:

- Maintain a healthy weight through diet and exercise, and avoid rapid weight loss.

Gallstones are more common in women, especially during pregnancy and menopause due to hormonal changes. By following a healthy diet, maintaining a healthy weight, and engaging in regular physical activity, women can reduce their risk of gallstones. Regular medical check-ups and discussing any gallbladder symptoms with a healthcare provider are crucial for early detection and management.

CHAPTER IV

HOW DIET AFFECTS GALLSTONE FORMATION IN WOMEN

Diet plays a pivotal role in the formation and management of gallstones, especially among women. Understanding this connection can help in making informed dietary choices to either prevent or manage gallstones. Several dietary factors are linked to gallstone formation, with distinct impacts based on their composition and consumption frequency.

Increased Risk Factors:

Women who consume diets high in refined sugars, sweetened foods, and fructose are at a greater risk of developing gallstones. Additionally, diets that are low in fiber and high in unhealthy fats—such as those found in fast food—exacerbate this risk. Low vitamin C intake further compounds the problem, as vitamin C plays a role in maintaining gallbladder health.

Protective Factors:

On the flip side, a diet rich in certain nutrients and foods can offer protection against gallstones. Monounsaturated fats found in olive oil and avocados, fiber from fruits, vegetables, and whole grains, and omega-3 fatty acids from fish like salmon all contribute to a healthier gallbladder. Moderate alcohol consumption and vitamin C supplementation are also beneficial in reducing the risk of gallstone formation.

Foods to Include

Incorporating specific foods into your diet can help manage and prevent gallstones. Focus on:

- Fruits and Vegetables: Aim to eat a variety of high-fiber fruits and vegetables daily. Apples, citrus fruits, bell peppers, and leafy greens are especially beneficial.

- Fiber-Rich Foods: Incorporate beans, lentils, whole grains, and nuts. These foods promote healthy digestion and reduce gallbladder disease risk.

- Low-Fat Dairy: Choose low-fat or fat-free dairy products to lower dietary fat intake and ease the burden on your gallbladder.

- Lean Proteins: Opt for lean proteins like poultry, fish, and plant-based options such as tofu and beans. These are less taxing on the gallbladder compared to high-fat meats.

Foods to Avoid

To minimize the risk of gallstone formation, limit or avoid the following:

- Sugary Foods: Cut back on foods high in refined sugars and fructose, as they can increase gallstone risk.

- High-Fat Foods: Avoid saturated fats found in butter, cheese, and fatty cuts of meat.

Replace these with healthier fats like olive oil and avocados.

- Fast Foods: Limit intake of fast foods, which are often high in unhealthy fats and low in essential nutrients.

By following these guidelines and focusing on a balanced, nutrient-rich diet, women can better manage their gallbladder health and reduce the likelihood of gallstone formation.

NOURISHING BREAKFAST RECIPES FOR GALLSTONE IN WOMEN

Blueberry Energy Bites

INGREDIENTS

for 4 servings

1 cup dry oat(100 g)

¼ cup almond butter(60 g)

¼ cup honey(85 g)

½ cup dried blueberry(50 g)

¼ teaspoon cinnamon

½ teaspoon vanilla

salt, optional

INSTRUCTIONS

Mix oats, almond butter and honey in a large bowl.

Add dried blueberries, cinnamon, vanilla, and salt and mix to combine.

Place bowl in the refrigerator for 30-60 minutes, or until the mixture has solidified.

Mold mixture into bite-sized balls.

Serve immediately.

Gluten-Free Dough Biscuits

INGREDIENTS

for 12 servings

1 cup full-fat greek yogurt(285 g)

2 cups gluten-free flour blend(250 g), plus more for flouring

2 teaspoons baking powder

salt, as desired

2 tablespoons butter, melted

INSTRUCTIONS

Preheat oven to 425°F (220°C).

In a large bowl, mix together the yogurt, gluten-free flour blend, baking powder, and salt until a dough forms.

Transfer the dough to a lightly-floured surface and flatten into a 12-inch (30-cm) disk.

Use a small cookie cutter to punch out 12 biscuit rounds.

Transfer the rounds to a parchment-lined baking sheet.

Use a pastry brush to brush the butter on the biscuits and lightly sprinkle the tops with salt.

Bake for 15 minutes, until the biscuits are set and just starting to brown.

Enjoy!

Apple Cinnamon Instant Oatmeal

INGREDIENTS

for 1 serving

½ cup instant oatmeal(50 g)

3 tablespoons freeze-dried apple, chopped

1 tablespoon pecan, chopped

1 tablespoon cinnamon

⅛ teaspoon vanilla bean

2 teaspoons sugar, of choice

¾ cup water(175 mL), or milk, boiled

INSTRUCTIONS

Add the instant oatmeal, freeze-dried apples, pecans, cinnamon, vanilla bean, and sugar into a mason jar.

Store in a cool, dry place for up to a month.

To prepare, pour boiling water or milk over oats. Stir to combine and let sit for 3 minutes.

Serve with fresh chopped apples. Enjoy!

Roti Jala

INGREDIENTS

for 6 servings

2 cups flour(250 g)

1 cup water(240 mL)

1 cup coconut milk(240 mL)

2 eggs

1 teaspoon salt

1 teaspoon turmeric

vegetable oil, as needed

SPECIAL EQUIPMENT

1 plastic water bottle

1 sharp pointed knife

INSTRUCTIONS

In a medium bowl, whisk together the flour, water, coconut milk, eggs, salt, and turmeric until smooth. (If any clumps remain, run mixture through a sieve.)

Using a sharp-pointed knife (a corkscrew or nail works just as well), poke three holes in the cap of a plastic water bottle.

Fill the bottle with your pancake batter.

Heat a very lightly greased nonstick skillet over medium heat. Working quickly, invert the water bottle and drizzle the batter in quick circular motions forming a netlike pattern.

Allow the pancake to cook for one to two minutes. Do not flip and watch closely so it doesn't burn.

Remove from pan, fold in the sides, and roll up. Serve with curry.

Loaded Breakfast Sweet Potato

INGREDIENTS

for 1 serving

1 sweet potato, small

2 tablespoons almond butter

½ slice banana, sliced

1 tablespoon almond, roasted, unsalted, and chopped

1 tablespoon blueberry

1 teaspoon honey

INSTRUCTIONS

Using a fork, poke holes on the top of the sweet potato.

Microwave on high for 10 minutes, or until the potato can be easily pierced with a knife.

Gently slice the sweet potato in half, lengthwise, and spread almond butter on each side. Top with banana slices, almonds, and blueberries, and drizzle with honey.

Almond Milk

INGREDIENTS

for 4 servings

1 cup raw almond(140 g)

1 tablespoon vanilla extract

3 tablespoons honey

1 pinch salt

6 cups water(1.5 L)

INGREDIENTS

for 4 servings

1 cup raw almond(140 g)

1 tablespoon vanilla extract

3 tablespoons honey

1 pinch salt

6 cups water(1.5 L)

INSTRUCTIONS

In a medium bowl, soak 1 cup of raw almonds in 2 cups (.5 L) of water overnight.

Drain the bowl of water and place the almonds in a blender.

Add 1 tablespoon vanilla, 3 tablespoons honey, 1 pinch of salt, and 4 cups (1 L) of water to the blender.

Blend the mixture on high for 90 seconds.

Use a cheesecloth to strain the liquid into a pouring container.

(Optional) refrigerate 1-2 hours or serve immediately.

Enjoy!

Tropical Coconut Smoothie Bowl

INGREDIENTS

for 1 serving

¼ cup coconut milk(60 g)

½ cup mango(80 g), peeled and cubed

½ cup pineapple(80 g), peeled and cubed

½ cup ice(110 g)

topping of your choice

INSTRUCTIONS

Add all the ingredients to a blender and mix on high.

Pour into a bowl or half a coconut, and top with desired fruit and other toppings.

Enjoy!

Bean And Cheese Toaster "Quesadilla"

INGREDIENTS

for 1 serving

1 large flour tortilla

¼ cup refried beans(40 g)

5 slices jalapeño

¼ cup shredded cheese blend(25 g)

salsa, for serving

INSTRUCTIONS

Using a butter knife, spread the refried beans in an even layer onto the tortilla.

Add the jalapeño slices and shredded cheese to the top half of the tortilla.

Fold the tortilla in half from the bottom, then fold in the sides, being careful not to tear the tortilla.

Toast on medium-high, until golden brown. Watch to make sure it doesn't burn. Let cool for 1-2 minutes before removing from the toaster.

Serve with salsa, if desired.

Enjoy!

Lower-Carb Biscuits And Gravy

INGREDIENTS

for 6 servings

BISCUITS

2 cups almond flour(190 g)

1 tablespoon baking powder

salt

½ cup plain greek yogurt(140 g)

2 large eggs

2 tablespoons honey

GRAVY

oil, of choice, for cooking

1 lb lean sausage(455 g), or ground turkey

¼ cup almond flour(25 g)

¼ teaspoon cayenne

¼ teaspoon paprika

½ tablespoon fresh rosemary, chopped

½ tablespoon fresh sage, chopped

salt, to taste

pepper, to taste

2 cups milk(480 mL), of choice

INSTRUCTIONS

Preheat the oven to 350°F (180°C). Line a baking sheet with parchment paper.

Make the biscuits: In a medium bowl, add the almond flour, baking powder, and salt. Whisk to combine.

In a separate large bowl, add the Greek yogurt, eggs, and honey. Whisk to combine.

Sift the dry ingredients through a fine-mesh sieve into the wet ingredients. Mix to combine until fluffy. Do not overmix.

Using a large ice cream scoop or a large spoon, scoop dough onto the lined baking sheet, spacing evenly. You should have about 6 biscuits. (If the oven is not ready, keep biscuits in the refrigerator so that they do not spread out and flatten.)

Bake for 15-20 minutes, or until golden brown.

Make the gravy: Drizzle a bit of oil in a large skillet over medium-high heat, then add the sausage and cook 7-10 minutes, or until browned.

Reduce the heat to medium-low and add ¼ cup (25 g) of almond flour, the cayenne, paprika, rosemary, sage, salt, and pepper. Stir to combine, then add the milk.

Simmer the gravy until it reaches your desired consistency, stirring occasionally. You can add up to ¼ cup (25 g) more almond flour for a thicker, heartier gravy.

Serve the gravy hot, poured over a warm biscuit.

Tofu Scramble Breakfast Burrito

INGREDIENTS

for 4 servings

3 medium yukon potatoes, peeled and cubed

olive oil, to taste

½ teaspoon smoked paprika

½ teaspoon dried oregano

3 teaspoons garlic powder, divided

kosher salt, to taste

pepper, to taste

14 oz extra firm tofu(395 g), 1 block

3 tablespoons low sodium soy sauce

3 tablespoons nutritional yeast

1 teaspoon onion powder

½ teaspoon ground turmeric

1 cup grape tomatoes(150 g), halved

3 cups fresh spinach(120 g)

4 large flour tortillas

1 avocado, for serving, diced

hot sauce, for serving

INSTRUCTIONS

Preheat the oven to 400°F (200°C).

Add the potatoes to a baking sheet with a drizzle of olive oil, the paprika, oregano, ½ teaspoon of garlic powder, salt, and pepper and toss until well coated.

Bake for 20 minutes, flipping halfway through, until the potatoes are tender.

Heat a drizzle of olive oil in a large saucepan over medium heat. Once the oil begins to shimmer, crumble the block of tofu into the pan until it resembles the consistency of scrambled eggs, being careful not to over-crumble because it will continue to break apart as you cook. Cook for 4-5 minutes, until the tofu is slightly golden.

Add the soy sauce, nutritional yeast, the remaining 2½ teaspoons garlic powder, the onion powder, turmeric, salt, and pepper and stir until well combined. Add the tomatoes and cook for 4-5 minutes, until the tomatoes become slightly wrinkled. Add the spinach and cook until wilted, 3-4 minutes.

To assemble a burrito, add ¼ of the tofu scramble, ¼ of the potatoes, some avocado, and hot sauce to the center of a tortilla. Fold in the sides and roll up, keeping the filling tucked in place. Repeat with the remaining ingredients. Cut in half and serve.

Savory Vegetable Crostata

INGREDIENTS

for 8 servings

CRUST

¾ cup all purpose flour(95 g), plus more for dusting

¾ cup whole wheat flour(95 g)

½ teaspoon kosher salt

6 tablespoons unsalted butter, cubed and chilled

3 tablespoons cold water

FILLING

3 tablespoons olive oil, divided

6 cloves garlic, peeled and stems removed

1 large yellow onion, thinly sliced

1 ½ teaspoons kosher salt, divided

2 medium red potatoes, thinly sliced

⅓ cup water(80 mL)

¼ teaspoon red pepper flakes

2 rainbow swiss chards, stem and leaves separated, thinly sliced

8 oz goat cheese(225 g), room temperature

1 large egg, beaten

INSTRUCTIONS

Make the crust: In a large bowl, mix together the all-purpose flour, whole wheat flour, and salt. Add the butter and, using a pastry cutter, work it into the flour until only pea-sized pieces remain. Add the water, starting with 3 tablespoons, and mix the dough with your fingers until it is moist enough to hold together. Add more water as needed, 1 tablespoon at a time. Turn the dough onto a clean surface, form into a disc, and wrap with plastic wrap. Refrigerate for 30-60 minutes.

Preheat the oven to 375°F (190°C). Line a baking sheet with parchment paper.

While the dough is resting, make the filling: Add 2 tablespoons of olive oil and the garlic cloves to a large, high-walled skillet over medium heat. Cook for 3 minutes, until the garlic just begins to brown. Add the onion and ½ teaspoon of salt. Cook for 20-25 minutes, until the onion is caramelized. Remove from the pan and set aside to cool in a bowl. To the same pan, add the potatoes, ½ teaspoon of salt, and the water. Increase the heat to medium-high, cover, and cook for 3-5 minutes, until the potatoes are almost fully cooked and the water is nearly evaporated. Remove the lid and cook for 2 minutes more to completely evaporate the water. Remove potatoes from the pan and set aside to cool.

To the same pan, add the remaining tablespoon of olive oil, the red pepper flakes, and chard stems. Reduce the heat to medium and cook for 3 minutes, until the stems are softened. Add the chard leaves and remaining ½ teaspoon of salt and cook for 5 minutes, until wilted and reduced in volume by half. Remove the pan from the heat.

Remove the garlic cloves from the caramelized onions and transfer to a small bowl. Mash with the back of a fork, then add to the softened goat cheese and stir to combine.

Stir the onions into the pan with the sautéed chard.

Assemble the crostata: Roll the dough out on a lightly floured surface into a 12-inch (30 cm) wide circle, about ⅛ inch (3 mm) thick. Transfer the dough to the prepared baking sheet.

Spread ½ cup (110 G) of the garlic goat cheese over the center of the dough, leaving a 2-inch (50 cm) border around the edges. Arrange half of the potatoes, slightly overlapping, over the goat cheese, then top with half of the Swiss chard and onion mixture. Repeat with remaining potatoes and chard mixture.

Fold the edges of the crust up and over the filling to create a rustic look. Brush the crust with the beaten egg. Top with dollops of the remaining goat cheese.

Bake the crostata for 45-50 minutes, until the crust is golden brown.

Let cool for 10 minutes before slicing and serving.

Sweet Potato Breakfast Bake

INGREDIENTS

for 8 servings

2 large sweet potatoes

1 tablespoon olive oil

2 teaspoons salt, divided

2 teaspoons pepper, divided

8 eggs

1 tomato, diced

¼ cup green onion(40 g), chopped

1 bell pepper, diced and cooked

½ teaspoon garlic powder

½ cup milk(120 mL)

cooking spray

10 slices ham

2 cups spinach(80 g)

INSTRUCTIONS

Preheat the oven to 425°F (220°C).

Using a mandolin, slice the sweet potatoes lengthwise into about 3-millimeter thick slices.

In a large bowl, combine the sliced sweet potatoes, oil, 1 teaspoon of salt, and 1 teaspoon pepper. Toss until well coated.

Lay out sweet potato slices on a baking sheet and bake for 10 minutes, until the edges start to crisp.

In a large bowl, combine the eggs, tomatoes, green onions, bell pepper, garlic powder, remaining teaspoon of salt, remaining teaspoon of pepper, and the milk. Whisk well.

Remove sweet potatoes from the oven and reduce the oven temperature to 400°F (200°C) .

Grease a 9 x 5-inch (23 x 13 cm) loaf pan. Line the sides and base of the pan with sweet potato slices, overlapping slightly.

Layer half of the ham slices over the sweet potato, then add the spinach, another layer of sweet potato, the egg mixture, the rest of the ham, and the rest of the sweet potato slices.

Fold the outside sweet potato slices over the loaf.

Bake for 30 minutes.

Invert the loaf onto a serving plate, then slice and serve.

Spaghetti Squash Nests

INGREDIENTS

for 4 servings

1 medium spaghetti squash, about 2 1/3 or 3 pounds (1.1 or 1.3 grams)

½ cup water(120 mL)

1 cup grated parmesan cheese(110 g)

kosher salt, to taste

ground black pepper, to taste

4 large eggs

olive oil, cooking spray

2 tablespoons fresh herb, such as chives, thyme, or parsley - minced

INSTRUCTIONS

Preheat the oven to 350°F (180°C). Line a baking sheet with parchment paper.

Using a fork, poke holes lengthwise around the center of the spaghetti squash.

Microwave for 2 minutes.

Cut the ends off of the squash, then slice in half lengthwise. Remove the seeds and pulp.

Place half of the squash flesh-side down in a microwave-safe dish with high sides. Pour ½ cup (120 ML) of water over the top of the squash and microwave on high for 3 minutes, or when a fork easily pulls the squash away from the skin in long strands that look like spaghetti. Repeat with second half— there will still be water left over from the first half. Cool the squash until it can be safely handled, about 10 minutes.

Use a fork to remove all of the squash from the skin, breaking it up into small strands. You should have approximately 4 cups of squash (820 G). Transfer to a medium bowl and stir in the Parmesan cheese, salt, and pepper.

Divide the squash into 4 1-cup (205 G each cup) (2 portions and place on the prepared baking sheet. Shape into nests, creating a well large enough to fit an egg in the center of each.

Bake for 10 minutes, until the squash is starting to brown. Remove from the oven and let cool for 5 minutes.

Crack the eggs into a small bowl, 1 at a time, then pour into the wells of the squash nests. Season with salt and pepper.

Bake for 12-15 minutes, depending on your preferred doneness for the eggs.

Garnish each nest with fresh herbs and serve.

NOURISHING LUNCH RECIPES FOR GALLSTONE IN WOMEN

Noodle Broth For One

INGREDIENTS

200ml vegetable stock made from 1/2 cube of reduced salt stock cube

2cm/1 inch root ginger, grated

1 red chilli, finely chopped, seeds removed

1 spring onion, finely chopped

1 tbsp sesame oil

1/2 tbsp reduced salt soy sauce

50g tofu diced

½ pak choi, chopped or shredded

50g rice noodles

To garnish, 1 tbsp chopped fresh coriander & lime wedge

INSTRUCTIONS

Bring the vegetable stock to simmer in a saucepan and then add the ginger, spring onion, pak choi, sesame oil and soy sauce.

After 5 minutes add the tofu, noodles and chilli and stir. Take off the heat and leave for 5 minutes to allow to cook through.

Serve with the fresh coriander and lime wedge on top.

Crusted Salmon Fillets

INGREDIENTS

2 salmon fillets, skin removed

40g wholemeal bread crumbs

3 teaspoons pesto, we used basil pesto

1 teaspoon rapeseed oil

INSTRUCTIONS

Spread one teaspoon of the pesto on the top of the salmon fillets.

Mix the breadcrumbs with the remaining pesto.

Carefully place the breadcrumb mixture on top of the salmon fillets. It should stick to the pesto topping.

Heat the grill to a moderate heat.

Gently warm the oil in a non-stick frying pan, that is oven proof.

Use a pallet knife to pick up the fillets and carefully place them in the pan.

Cook on a moderate heat for about 4-5 minutes.

Cook for a further 3-5 minutes under the grill taking care to ensure that the top does not burn.

Serve with green vegetables and with new potatoes or puy lentils or a green salad.

Sausage and Peppers Soup

INGREDIENTS

2 tablespoon olive oil

16 ounce cooked smoked sausage, halved lengthwise and sliced

4 red, yellow, green, and/or orange sweet peppers, cut into bite-size strips

2 cup chopped onions

4 cloves garlic, minced

2 14.5 ounce cans diced tomatoes with basil, garlic, and oregano, undrained

1 6 ounce can tomato paste

½ teaspoon crushed red pepper

8 cup reduced-sodium chicken broth

½ cup chopped fresh basil

Salt and black pepper

INSTRUCTIONS

In a 4- to 5-qt. Dutch oven heat oil over medium-high. Add sausage; cook and stir 2 to 3 minutes or until browned. Remove sausage. Add sweet peppers, onions, and garlic to Dutch oven. Cook and stir 4 to 5 minutes or until tender and starting to brown. Remove from heat. Stir in sausage, tomatoes, tomato paste, and crushed red pepper.

Divide sausage mixture between two freezer containers or bags. Label and freeze up to 3 months.

To serve, thaw one container of sausage mixture in refrigerator 1 to 2 days (mixture may still be a bit icy). Transfer to a 4- to 5-qt. Dutch oven. Add 4 cups of the broth. Cook over medium heat until heated through, stirring occasionally. Stir in 1/4 cup of the basil. Season to taste with salt and black pepper.

Slow Cooker

Thaw one container of sausage mixture as directed. Transfer to a 3 1/2- or 4-qt. slow cooker. Stir in 4 cups of the broth. Cover and cook on low 5 to 6 hours or high 2 1/2 to 3 hours. Stir in 1/4 cup of the basil. Season to taste with salt and black pepper.

Spicy Chicken Pitta Pockets

INGREDIENTS

2 tbsp Greek Style low-fat yogurt

2 tsp harissa paste

1 tbsp olive oil

1 small onion

1 large chicken breast fillet, skin removed and cut into slices

1 red pepper, de-seeded and sliced

100g mushrooms, sliced

2 wholemeal pitta breads

Salad leaves, washed and dried

Two lemon quarters – optional

INSTRUCTIONS

Toast the pitta breads, when ready they should puff up. Slice along the top edge to form a pocket which you can fill later with the chicken mixture and salad.

Meanwhile, cook the onion gently in the oil for a few minutes until softened.

Add the sliced chicken and cook until brown on all sides

Add the mushrooms and peppers and continue to cook for another 5-10 minutes until the mushrooms are soft and the peppers are softening but still have some crunch. Stir in the harissa paste, making sure that all the chicken and vegetables are coated. Allow to cool a little.

Now you need to assemble the contents. Start but putting a layer of salad into each pitta followed by the chicken mixture. Finnish with a layer of salad leaves and a drizzle of yogurt.

Serve immediately with lemon quarters

Recipe Tip

You can use the same combination in sandwiches or wraps. Choose wholemeal varieties.

Tasty Tuna Sandwiches

INGREDIENTS

1 can of tuna in spring water, drained

2 tbsp low fat Greek style yogurt

1 tbsp chopped fresh coriander

Ground black pepper

4 slices wholemeal bread or 2 rolls

1/4 cucumber, diced

1/4 red bell pepper, diced

handful fresh salad leaves

Scrape low fat mayonnaise - if needed

INSTRUCTIONS

Mix with the yogurt with the coriander and season with black pepper. Flake in the tuna and add the diced cucumber and red pepper.

Spread the 2 slices of bread with a little low-fat mayonnaise (to help the filling stick to the bread) and then divide the tuna mixture over the slices.

Top the filling with salad leaves and the remaining bread slices and serve.

Tuna Beetroot Avocado and Walnut Salad

INGREDIENTS

3 ripe avocados

6 (480g) whole beetroots, cooked & ready to eat (not in vinegar)

3 small tins of tuna in water, about 210g tuna meat

3 clementines, segmented

120g walnuts/walnut pieces

3 tbsp extra virgin olive oil

6 tbsp good quality balsamic vinegar

Handful of basil leaves

INSTRUCTIONS

Peel and slice the avocados, slice the beetroots and display them around the plate or salad bowl.

Roughly chop the walnuts and sprinkle these over the avocado and beets along with the tuna and Clementine segments.

In a jug, whisk together the olive oil and balsamic vinegar and drizzle over the salad. Finish by decorating the top with some basil leaves.

Warming Tomato Soup

INGREDIENTS

2 tablespoons Sunflower or Olive oil

700g ripe Cherry Tomatoes, halved

1 Fennel bulb, thinly sliced

1 Onion, chopped

2 Garlic Cloves, crushed

2 teaspoons Sugar

2 small Potatoes – roughly diced

2 tablespoons White Wine Vinegar (30ml)

2 tablespoons Tomato Puree

2 tablespoons Sun Dried Tomatoes

1 litre Water

Black pepper

To Serve

60 ml Low Fat Greek Yogurt

A few fresh chives

INSTRUCTIONS

Cook the onion, garlic, potato and about 1/2 the fennel in the oil (without colouring) for about 5 minutes, or until softened.

Stir in the sugar and wine vinegar and continue to cook for a further 3-4 minutes.

Add the tomatoes, tomato puree, sun-dried tomatoes and cook for a further 5 minutes.

Add the water, bring to boiling point, then turn the heat low and simmer for 15-20 minutes.

Blend the soup using a stick blender.

Add the remaining thinly sliced fennel and cook for 10 minutes.

Serve with crusty bread, a swirl of low-fat Greek yoghurt and a few snipped chives.

Air Fryer Baked Potatoes

INGREDIENTS

2 large russet potatoes, scrubbed

1 tablespoon peanut oil

½ teaspoon coarse sea salt

INSTRUCTIONS

Gather all ingredients and preheat an air fryer to 400 degrees F (200 degrees C).

Brush potatoes with peanut oil, sprinkle with salt, and place them in the air fryer basket.

Cook potatoes until very tender when pierced with a fork, about 1 hour. Serve and enjoy!

Delicious Mediterranean Soup

INGREDIENTS

1 onion, finely chopped

1 clove garlic, crushed

1 tbsp olive oil

1 bell pepper (red or yellow), diced

2 courgettes, diced

1 tsp paprika

1 tsp fresh rosemary, chopped

1 tsp Balsamic vinegar

400g can chopped or pureed tomatoes

1-litre vegetable stock made from 2 low salt stock cubes

1 tbsp Tomato puree

1 sprig fresh flat-leaf parsley (optional)

Freshly ground pepper

INSTRUCTIONS

Heat the oil in a pan and gently cook the onion and garlic for 5 minutes without colouring.

Set aside 1 tbsp of diced pepper then add the remainder of the pepper along with the courgettes, paprika, rosemary to the pan and cook for a few minutes.

Add the balsamic vinegar, after 2 minutes add the tomatoes and stock and bring to the boil.

Gently simmer until the vegetables are cooked through and tender, about 10 minutes.

Finally, stir in the tomato paste. Either leave the soup as a rustic, chunky vegetable broth or use a handheld blender to blend until smooth.

Season with fresh ground pepper and serve topped with the reserved diced pepper and a sprig of parsley.

Cheese and Walnut Butties

INGREDIENTS

2 slices wholemeal, granary or rye bread

30g low-fat cheese spread such as Philadelphia

3 walnuts finely chopped

¼ stick celery, finely diced

Black pepper

INSTRUCTIONS

Spread the cheese evenly on both slices of bread. Season with black pepper.

Sprinkle the walnuts and sliced celery on top of one slice of bread.

Place the other slice on top, quarter and serve

Dukkah-crusted halloumi salad

INGREDIENTS

100g lettuce, shredded

1 large spring onion, thinly sliced

2 tomatoes, chopped

1/8 cucumber, chopped

70g cooked beetroot, chopped

4 radishes, sliced

75g light halloumi cheese, chopped into 2cm cubes

2 tsp Dukkah

For the dressing

2 level tbsp mango chutney

½ tsp white wine vinegar

6 drops of Tabasco sauce

INSTRUCTIONS

Pre-heat the grill. Line a grill pan with foil.

Divide the lettuce, spring onion, tomatoes, cucumber, beetroot and radishes between two plates.

Mix together the chopped halloumi and Dukkah in a bowl.

Transfer the coated halloumi and any excess Dukkah into the grill pan. Cook under the grill for a couple of minutes, turning once, until the Dukkah is lightly toasted.

Remove and add to the salad vegetables.

Heat a small saucepan over a medium heat, quickly add the mango chutney, white wine vinegar, tabasco and 40mls of water. Bubble for 20 to 30 seconds. You may need a little more vinegar depending on which brand of mango chutney you use. Pour the dressing over the salad and eat immediately.

NOURISHING DINNER RECIPES FOR GALLSTONE IN WOMEN

Savory Mexican Fish Tacos

INGREDIENTS

200g pack of fish goujons

1 tsp chipotle paste or harissa (add more for extra spice)

6 tbsp low fat natural yoghurt

4 soft corn tortillas

175g red and white cabbage, finely shredded

4 vine tomatoes, chopped

good handful chopped coriander

1 small red onion, finely chopped or sliced

juice 1 small lime, plus wedges to serve (optional)

INSTRUCTIONS

Heat the oven to 220C/ 200C fan/ Gas 7. Place the goujons on a baking sheet and bake for 12-15 mins, or according to pack instructions, until crispy. Meanwhile, mix the chipotle or harissa into the yoghurt, and warm the tortillas – they are best warmed over a gas flame.

To make the salad, toss the cabbage, coriander, tomatoes and onion with the lime juice.

Spread the tortillas with a little spicy yoghurt, then place the salad and fish down the centre. Top with a little more yoghurt, then fold and eat with your fingers. Serve with lime wedges.

Winter Vegetable Mulligatawny Soup

INGREDIENTS

3 tablespoons extra-virgin olive oil, divided

1 medium onion, finely chopped

2 medium carrots, finely chopped

1 medium parsnip, peeled and finely chopped

4 cups peeled diced acorn squash or butternut squash

1 medium green apple, peeled and finely chopped

1 tablespoon curry powder

3 cloves garlic, minced, divided

1 teaspoon grated fresh ginger

4 cups low-sodium vegetable broth

1 (14 ounce) can no-salt-added diced tomatoes

½ cup red lentils, picked over and rinsed

2 whole-wheat naan flatbreads, halved

¼ cup chopped fresh cilantro, plus more for garnish

INSTRUCTIONS

Preheat oven to 375°F. Line a baking sheet with foil.

Heat 2 tablespoons oil in a large saucepan over medium heat until shimmering. Add onion, carrots and parsnip and cook until the onions are translucent, about 6 minutes. Add squash, apple, curry powder, 2 cloves garlic and ginger and cook, stirring, until fragrant, 1 to 2 minutes. Add broth, tomatoes and lentils and stir to combine. Bring to a boil. Reduce heat to maintain a low simmer, cover and cook until the squash and lentils are tender, about 20 minutes.

Meanwhile, brush one side of each naan with the remaining 1 tablespoon oil. Sprinkle with the remaining 1 clove garlic and place on the prepared baking sheet. Bake until warmed, 5 to 6 minutes. Remove from oven and sprinkle with cilantro.

Gently mash some of the soup with a potato masher to achieve desired consistency. (Alternatively, transfer half the soup to a blender and puree. Use caution when blending hot liquids.) Garnish the soup with cilantro and serve with the naan.

Beer-Battered Fish Tacos with Tomato & Avocado Salsa for Two

INGREDIENTS

Tomato & Avocado Salsa

1 large tomato, diced

¼ cup diced red onion

½ jalapeno, minced

2-3 tablespoons lime juice

¼ teaspoon kosher salt

⅛ teaspoon freshly ground pepper

½ avocado, diced

¼ cup chopped fresh cilantro

Pinch of cayenne, if desired

Fish Tacos

3 tablespoons all-purpose flour

⅛ teaspoon ground cumin

⅛ teaspoon salt

⅛ teaspoon cayenne pepper, or to taste

⅓ cup beer

8 ounces tilapia fillet, cut crosswise into 1-inch wide strips

2 teaspoons canola oil

4 corn tortillas, warmed (see Tip)

INSTRUCTIONS

To prepare salsa: Combine tomato, onion, jalapeno, lime juice to taste, kosher salt and pepper in a medium bowl. Stir in avocado and cilantro. Add cayenne (if using).

To prepare tacos: Combine flour, cumin, salt and cayenne in a medium bowl. Whisk in beer to create a batter.

Coat tilapia pieces in the batter. Heat oil in a large nonstick skillet over medium-high heat. Letting excess batter drip back into the bowl, add the fish to the pan; cook until crispy and golden, 2 to 4 minutes per side. Serve the fish with tortillas and the salsa.

Savory Tomatillo Salad

INGREDIENTS

1 ¼ pounds salmon fillet, cut into 4 portions

2 tablespoons extra-virgin olive oil, divided

¾ teaspoon kosher salt, divided

½ teaspoon ground pepper, divided

½ teaspoon ground cumin

8 ounces tomatillos, husked, rinsed and chopped (see Tip)

1 medium tomato, chopped

½ cup chopped fresh cilantro

½ cup chopped red onion

1 medium jalapeño pepper, chopped

2 tablespoons lime juice

INSTRUCTIONS

Position rack in upper third of oven; preheat broiler to high.

Place salmon on a rimmed baking sheet. Drizzle with 1 tablespoon oil and sprinkle with 1/2 teaspoon salt, 1/4 teaspoon pepper and cumin. Broil the salmon until it is opaque and flakes easily with a fork, 6 to 9 minutes.

Meanwhile, combine tomatillos, tomato, cilantro, onion, jalapeño and lime juice with the remaining 1 tablespoon oil and 1/4 teaspoon each salt and pepper in a medium bowl. Serve the salmon with the salad.

Tips

Tip: Although you'll want to remove the husk (and rinse off the sticky coating) before eating, look for firm tomatillos with an intact husk that's tight to the fruit.

Chicken & Mushroom Ragu

INGREDIENTS

1 28-ounce can no-salt-added whole peeled tomatoes, preferably San Marzano

¼ cup extra-virgin olive oil

1 medium onion, chopped

2 medium carrots, chopped

8 ounces cremini mushrooms, quartered

1 ¾ pounds boneless, skinless chicken thighs, trimmed and cut into 1-inch pieces

2 cloves garlic, grated

¼ cup tomato paste

½ cup dry red wine

½ teaspoon salt

¼ teaspoon crushed red pepper

1 tablespoon chopped fresh rosemary

1 pound whole-wheat linguine or fettuccine

½ cup grated Romano cheese

½ cup chopped fresh parsley

INSTRUCTIONS

Put a large pot of water on to boil.

Pour tomatoes and their juice into a medium bowl. Using your hands, break the tomatoes into chunks.

Heat oil in an electric pressure cooker on Sauté mode. Add onion, carrots and mushrooms; cook, stirring, until the mushrooms have released their liquid, about 5 minutes. Add chicken, garlic and tomato paste. Cook, stirring occasionally, until the chicken is coated and the mixture at the bottom of the pan is beginning to brown, about 4 minutes. Add wine, salt, crushed red pepper and the tomatoes. Cook, scraping up the browned bits, until beginning to boil, about 2 minutes. Turn off the heat.

Close and lock the lid. Cook at High pressure for 10 minutes. Release the pressure manually. Stir in rosemary.

Meanwhile, cook pasta according to package directions. Drain and serve topped with the sauce, cheese and parsley.

To make ahead

Refrigerate ragu (Steps 2-4) for up to 3 days or freeze for up to 3 months.

Quinoa, Avocado & Chickpea Salad over Mixed Greens

INGREDIENTS

⅔ cup water

⅓ cup quinoa

¼ teaspoon kosher salt or other coarse salt

1 clove garlic, crushed and peeled

2 teaspoons grated lemon zest

3 tablespoons lemon juice

3 tablespoons olive oil

¼ teaspoon ground pepper

1 cup rinsed no-salt-added canned chickpeas

1 medium carrot, shredded (1/2 cup)

½ avocado, diced

1 (5 ounce) package prewashed mixed greens, such as spring mix or baby kale-spinach blend (8 cups packed)

INSTRUCTIONS

Bring water to a boil in a small saucepan. Stir in quinoa. Reduce heat to low, cover, and simmer until all the liquid is absorbed, about 15 minutes. Use a fork to fluff and separate the grains; let cool for 5 minutes.

Meanwhile, sprinkle salt over garlic on a cutting board. Mash the garlic with the side of a spoon until a paste forms. Scrape into a medium bowl. Whisk in lemon zest, lemon juice, oil, and pepper. Transfer 3 Tbsp. of the dressing to a small bowl and set aside.

Add chickpeas, carrot, and avocado to the bowl with the remaining dressing; gently toss to combine. Let stand for 5 minutes to allow flavors to blend. Add the quinoa and gently toss to coat.

Place greens in a large bowl and toss with the reserved 3 Tbsp. dressing. Divide the greens between 2 plates and top with the quinoa mixture.

Stuffed Sweet Potato with Hummus Dressing

`INGREDIENTS

1 large sweet potato, scrubbed

¾ cup chopped kale

1 cup canned black beans, rinsed

¼ cup hummus

2 tablespoons water

INSTRUCTIONS

Prick sweet potato all over with a fork. Microwave on High until cooked through, 7 to 10 minutes.

Meanwhile, wash kale and drain, allowing water to cling to the leaves. Place in a medium saucepan; cover and cook over medium-high heat, stirring once or twice, until wilted. Add beans; add a tablespoon or two of water if the pot is dry. Continue cooking, uncovered, stirring occasionally, until the mixture is steaming hot, 1 to 2 minutes.

Split the sweet potato open and top with the kale and bean mixture. Combine hummus and 2 tablespoons water in a small dish. Add additional water as needed to reach desired consistency. Drizzle the hummus dressing over the stuffed sweet potato.

Vegetables with Charred Lemon-Garlic Vinaigrette

INGREDIENTS

2 medium zucchini, trimmed and halved lengthwise

1 pound asparagus, trimmed

5 - 6 tablespoons Charred Lemon-Garlic Vinaigrette, divided

1 ¼ pounds salmon fillet, cut into 4 portions

¼ teaspoon salt, divided

¼ teaspoon ground pepper, divided

INSTRUCTIONS

Preheat grill to medium-high.

Brush zucchini and asparagus with 2 tablespoons vinaigrette and sprinkle with 1/8 teaspoon each salt and pepper. Drizzle salmon with 2 teaspoons vinaigrette and sprinkle with the remaining 1/8 teaspoon each salt and pepper.

Place the vegetables and the salmon pieces, skin-side down, on the grill. Grill the vegetables, turning a few times, until tender, 6 to 8 minutes. Grill the salmon, without turning, until it flakes with a fork, 8 to 10 minutes.

Cut the vegetables into 3 or 4 pieces and place in a medium bowl. Drizzle with 2 tablespoons vinaigrette and toss to coat. Remove the skin from the salmon, if desired; serve the salmon alongside the vegetables. Drizzle the salmon with 1 tablespoon vinaigrette, if desired. (Refrigerate any remaining vinaigrette for up to 3 days.)

Vegetarian Sliders with Black Beans, Chard & Poblanos

INGREDIENTS

1 cup boiling water

1 tablespoon honey

¾ teaspoon salt, divided

1 cup cider vinegar

1 small red onion, thinly sliced

3 medium poblano peppers

1 tablespoon extra-virgin olive oil, divided

1 medium yellow onion, diced

3 cloves garlic, minced

1 bunch chard, including stems, chopped (8 cups)

4 ½ cups cooked or canned (rinsed) black beans, patted dry

1 large egg, lightly beaten

½ cup fine dry whole-wheat breadcrumbs

2 teaspoons Creole seasoning, plus more for serving

Cooking spray

16 slider buns, preferably whole-wheat, split and toasted

1 cup crumbled feta cheese

INSTRUCTIONS

Combine boiling water, honey and 1/2 teaspoon salt in a heatproof bowl, stirring to dissolve the honey and salt. Stir in vinegar, then add red onion. Set aside.

Position rack in upper third of oven; preheat broiler to high. Place peppers on a baking sheet and broil, turning occasionally, until blackened on all sides, 12 to 15 minutes. Transfer to a bowl, cover with plastic wrap and let steam until cool enough to handle, about 15 minutes. Peel and seed the peppers. Slice or tear them into strips; set aside.

Meanwhile, heat 1 1/2 teaspoons oil in a large skillet over medium heat. Add yellow onion and cook, stirring occasionally, until soft and light golden brown, 3 to 5 minutes. Add garlic; cook, stirring occasionally, until fragrant and soft, 1 to 2 minutes. Scrape onto a plate.

Return the pan to medium heat and add the remaining 1 1/2 teaspoons oil and chard. Cook, stirring frequently and adding a splash of water if it starts to stick, until the stems are tender and any liquid has evaporated, 5 to 8 minutes. Scrape onto the plate and let cool, about 10 minutes.

Place beans in a large bowl and coarsely mash. Add the chard mixture, egg, breadcrumbs, Creole seasoning and the remaining 1/4 teaspoon salt; mix well.

Coat a baking sheet with cooking spray. Using about 1/3 cup to make each, portion the bean mixture into 16 patties, 1/2 inch thick, and place on the prepared baking sheet. Coat the patties lightly with cooking spray. Broil until browned and firm on top, 6 to 8 minutes. Flip the patties and coat the other side with cooking spray. Broil until browned, 4 to 6 minutes more.

Serve the patties in buns, topped with the reserved peppers, pickled onion and feta. Sprinkle with more Creole seasoning, if desired.

White Bean Soup with Pasta

INGREDIENTS

1 tablespoon extra-virgin olive oil

1 ½ cups frozen mirepoix (diced onion, celery and carrot)

2 cloves garlic, minced

1 teaspoon Italian seasoning

1 teaspoon salt

¼ teaspoon crushed red pepper

¼ teaspoon ground pepper

1 28-ounce can no-salt-added diced tomatoes

2 cups low-sodium no-chicken broth or chicken broth

1 15-ounce can low-sodium cannellini beans, rinsed

8 ounces small whole-wheat pasta, such as elbows

1 ½ cups frozen cut-leaf spinach

4 tablespoons grated Parmesan cheese

INSTRUCTIONS

Put a large saucepan of water on to boil.

Heat oil in a large pot over medium-high heat. Add mirepoix and cook, stirring, until softened, about 3 minutes. Add garlic, Italian seasoning, salt, crushed red pepper and ground pepper and cook, stirring, until fragrant, about 1 minute. Add tomatoes and their juices, broth and beans and bring to a boil. Reduce heat to maintain a lively simmer. Cover and cook, stirring occasionally, until the tomatoes begin to break down, about 10 minutes.

Meanwhile, cook pasta in the boiling water for 1 minute less than the package directions. Drain.

Stir spinach into the soup. Stir in the pasta just before serving. Serve topped with Parmesan.

Baked Halibut with Brussels Sprouts

INGREDIENTS

1 pound Brussels sprouts, trimmed and sliced

1 fennel bulb, trimmed and cut into strips

1 tablespoon plus 1 teaspoon olive oil, divided

½ teaspoon salt, divided

½ teaspoon ground pepper, divided

1 (1 pound) halibut fillet, cut into 4 portions

4 cloves garlic, minced, divided

3 tablespoons lemon juice

2 tablespoons unsalted butter, melted

2 cups cooked quinoa

¼ cup chopped sun-dried tomatoes

¼ cup chopped pitted Kalamata olives

2 tablespoons chopped fresh Italian parsley or fennel fronds

INSTRUCTIONS

Position racks in upper and lower thirds of oven; preheat to 400 degrees F.

Combine Brussels sprouts, fennel, 1 Tbsp. oil, and 1/4 tsp. each salt and pepper in a large bowl; toss to coat. Spread in a single layer on a large rimmed baking sheet. Bake, stirring occasionally, until tender, 20 to 25 minutes.

Meanwhile, place halibut on another large rimmed baking sheet and top with half of the garlic and the remaining 1/4 tsp. each salt and pepper. Combine lemon juice and melted butter in a small bowl. Drizzle or brush half of the mixture over the fish. Bake until the fish is opaque and flakes easily with a fork, 12 to 15 minutes.

Meanwhile, combine quinoa, the remaining 1 tsp. oil, sun-dried tomatoes, olives, and parsley (or fennel fronds) in a medium bowl.

Add the remaining garlic to the lemon-butter mixture. Pour the mixture over the vegetables and bake for 1 minute more. Serve the halibut and vegetables alongside the quinoa mixture.

Chickpea & Potato Curry

INGREDIENTS

1 pound Yukon Gold potatoes, peeled and cut into 1-inch pieces

3 tablespoons grapeseed oil or canola oil

1 large onion, diced

3 cloves garlic, minced

2 teaspoons curry powder

¾ teaspoon salt

¼ teaspoon cayenne pepper

1 (14 ounce) can no-salt-added diced tomatoes

¾ cup water, divided

1 (15 ounce) can low-sodium chickpeas, rinsed

1 cup frozen peas

½ teaspoon garam masala (see Tip)

INSTRUCTIONS

Bring 1 inch of water to a boil in a large pot fitted with a steamer basket. Add potatoes, cover and steam until tender, 6 to 8 minutes. Set the potatoes aside. Dry the pot.

Heat oil in the pot over medium-high heat. Add onion and cook, stirring often, until soft and translucent, 3 to 5 minutes. Add garlic, curry powder, salt and cayenne; cook, stirring constantly, for 1 minute. Stir in tomatoes and their juice; cook for 2 minutes. Transfer the mixture to a blender or food processor. Add 1/2 cup water and puree until smooth.

Return the puree to the pot. Pulse the remaining 1/4 cup water in the blender or food processor to rinse the sauce residue. Add to the pot along with the reserved potatoes, chickpeas, peas and garam masala. Cook, stirring often, until hot, about 5 minutes.

Tips

Tip: Garam masala, a mix of coriander, black pepper, cumin, cardamom, cinnamon and other spices, adds a warming, complex layer of flavor to this Indian stew.

SNACKS, SALAD, DESSERT RECIPES FOR GALLSTONE IN WOMEN

Quick and Easy Jackfruit Salad Sandwiches

INGREDIENTS

2 10.6-oz. pkg. unseasoned shredded young jackfruit (see tip, recipe intro)

1 medium apple, chopped

¾ cup coarsely shredded carrots

½ cup chopped fresh parsley or cilantro

¼ cup chopped walnuts, toasted

1 teaspoon lemon zest

1 15-oz. can no-salt-added white beans, rinsed and drained (1½ cups)

¾ cup unsweetened, unflavored plant-based milk

1 medium avocado, halved, seeded, peeled, and thinly sliced

3 tablespoons lemon juice

4 teaspoons coarse ground mustard

2 cloves garlic, minced

½ teaspoon sea salt

4 whole grain English muffins, split and toasted

4 to 8 green or red leaf lettuce leaves, torn

2 medium tomatoes, each cut into 8 slices

Freshly ground black pepper

INSTRUCTIONS

Pat the jackfruit dry, if needed, using a clean kitchen towel or paper towels. In a large bowl toss together jackfruit and the next five ingredients (through lemon zest). Stir in ¾ cup of the beans.

In a blender or small food processor combine the remaining beans, the milk, one-fourth of the avocado, the lemon juice, mustard, garlic, and salt. Cover and blend until smooth, scraping sides as needed. Add blended bean mixture to jackfruit mixture. Toss to combine.

Top all eight English muffin halves with lettuce and tomatoes. Spoon jackfruit mixture over top. Add the remaining avocado slices and sprinkle with pepper. Serve immediately.

Savory Cherry Panna Cotta Parfaits

INGREDIENTS

¾ cup rolled oats

1 tablespoon chopped walnuts

3 Medjool dates, pitted and coarsely chopped

Pinch sea salt

2¼ cups unsweetened, unflavored plant milk

¼ cup cornstarch

3 tablespoons pure maple syrup

2 tablespoons lemon juice

1 teaspoon pure vanilla extract

½ teaspoon pure almond extract

2 cups fresh sweet cherries, pitted and halved (10 oz.)

¼ cup low- or no-sugar cherry preserves

2 tablespoons orange juice

INSTRUCTIONS

Preheat oven to 350°F. Place oats and walnuts on a parchment-lined baking sheet. Bake 10 minutes or until lightly toasted and starting to crisp. Cool on a wire rack about 5 minutes. In a small food processor combine oats mixture, dates, and salt. Cover and pulse to fine crumbs. Transfer to a small bowl. Drizzle with 1 tablespoon water and toss with a fork until mixture starts to cling together. Spoon into six half-pint glass jars; press with back of spoon to pack lightly.

In a medium saucepan whisk together milk, cornstarch, maple syrup, and 1 tablespoon of the lemon juice. Bring to boiling over medium-high. Boil 1 minute or until thickened, stirring frequently. Remove from heat and stir in extracts. Let cool 5 minutes. Pour into jars.

In a medium saucepan combine cherries, cherry preserves, orange juice, and the remaining 1 tablespoon lemon juice. Heat just until bubbling around the edges. Carefully spoon cherry mixture over pudding layer. Refrigerate at least 2 hours or overnight.

Delicious Harissa Cauliflower Steaks with Date Couscous

INGREDIENTS

¼ cup low-sodium vegetable broth

2 tablespoons lemon juice

1 tablespoon reduced-sodium soy sauce

2 teaspoons salt-free harissa seasoning

1¼ teaspoon sea salt

One 2¼ - to 2¾-lb. head cauliflower, trimmed and cut vertically into four 1½-inch-thick steaks

1 cup chopped onion

½ cup chopped pitted dates

½ cup chopped fresh cilantro

1 teaspoon ground cumin

½ teaspoon ground coriander

¼ teaspoon crushed red pepper

2 cups dry whole wheat pearl couscous

Lemon wedges

INSTRUCTIONS

In a small bowl whisk together broth, lemon juice, soy sauce, harissa seasoning, and ¼ teaspoon of the salt. Brush cauliflower steaks with broth mixture. Grill steaks, covered, over medium-high 12 to 15 minutes or until steaks are tender and lightly charred, turning and brushing with additional broth mixture once.

In a large saucepan combine onion, dates, ¼ cup of the cilantro, the cumin, coriander, crushed red pepper, the remaining 1 teaspoon salt, and 3 cups water. Bring to boiling. Stir in couscous; cover. Remove from heat and let stand 5 minutes. Toss to combine.

Serve cauliflower steaks with couscous. Sprinkle with the remaining ¼ cup cilantro. Serve with lemon wedges.

10-Minute Strawberry Cucumber Salad

INGREDIENTS

2 cups sliced fresh strawberries

1 cup halved cherry tomatoes

1 cup fresh mint leaves, chopped

1 cucumber, sliced

1 cup mixed greens

½ of a red onion, thinly sliced

½ cup walnuts, crushed

3 tablespoons orange juice

2 tablespoons Dijon mustard

1 tablespoon pure maple syrup

1 tablespoon apple cider vinegar

INSTRUCTIONS

In a large bowl combine the first seven ingredients (through walnuts); toss to combine.

For dressing, in a small bowl whisk together the remaining ingredients and 2 tablespoons water. Pour over salad; toss to coat. Serve immediately.

Delicious Plum Pasta Salad with Roasted Garlic Vinaigrette

INGREDIENTS

1 head garlic (2-inch diameter)

12 oz. dried whole wheat penne or rotini pasta

¼ cup red wine vinegar

1 teaspoon dried oregano, crushed

Sea salt, to taste

Freshly ground black pepper, to taste

1 15-oz. can no-salt-added butter beans, rinsed and drained (1½ cups)

1 cup chopped fresh plums

1½ cups Spicy Pickled Green Beans, chopped

1 2-oz. jar chopped pimientos, drained

¼ cup chopped fresh dill or ½ cup chopped fresh flat-leaf parsley

INSTRUCTIONS

Preheat oven to 400°F. Cut the top ¼ inch off garlic head so tops of cloves are exposed. Wrap head in foil. Roast 40 to 50 minutes or until very soft. Let cool. Squeeze garlic from papery skin into a large bowl and mash.

Meanwhile, cook pasta according to package directions. Reserve ¼ cup cooking water. Drain pasta. Rinse with cold water; drain again.

For dressing, add the ¼ cup pasta cooking water, the vinegar, and oregano to bowl with garlic; whisk until smooth. Season with salt and pepper.

Add pasta and the remaining ingredients to dressing. Toss to combine. Chill until ready to serve.

Classic Arugula and Peach Smoothie Bowls

INGREDIENTS

2 cups fresh baby arugula

⅔ cup orange juice

½ to ⅔ cup unsweetened, unflavored plant milk

1 teaspoon pure maple syrup

5 cups frozen chopped or sliced peaches

1 banana, sliced and frozen (¾ cup)

1 fresh peach, pitted and sliced

¾ cup fresh raspberries

2 tablespoons coarsely chopped roasted pistachios

2 tablespoons coarsely chopped toasted walnuts

INSTRUCTIONS

In a blender place arugula, orange juice, ½ cup of the milk, the maple syrup, frozen peaches, and banana in the order given. Cover and blend until smooth, stirring occasionally, adding additional milk if needed to reach desired consistency. Pour into bowls. Top with remaining ingredients.

Spicy Pickled Green Beans

INGREDIENTS

14 cloves garlic, lightly crushed

7 to 14 heads fresh dill or 1 to 2 teaspoons dill seeds (see tip in intro)

Crushed red pepper

4 lb. fresh green beans

4 cups white vinegar

4 cups water

¼ cup pure cane sugar

3 tablespoons sea salt

INSTRUCTIONS

Divide garlic and dill among seven sterilized pint jars. Add ⅛ teaspoon crushed red pepper to each jar. Trim beans as needed to fit in the jars. Pack beans upright in jars, placing together as tightly as you can; leave ½-inch headspace.

In a large saucepan combine the remaining ingredients. Bring to boiling. Add to jars, making sure to cover beans. Add lids to jars. Let cool on a wire rack. Let beans pickle in the refrigerator at least 1 week before serving. Store in the refrigerator up to 3 weeks.

Vegetarian Antipasto Salad

INGREDIENTS

1 2-inch garlic bulb + 1 clove garlic, minced

1 12-oz. package frozen artichoke hearts, thawed and halved

2 cups round red radishes, halved

2 kohlrabi, peeled and cut into ¼-inch-thick strips

½ cup + 1 tablespoon white balsamic vinegar

½ teaspoon sea salt

½ teaspoon freshly ground black pepper

2 cups low-sodium vegetable broth or water

1 cup dry pearled farro (see tip, recipe intro)

1 cup fresh basil

2 teaspoons Dijon mustard

1 15-oz. can no-salt-added butter beans or cannellini beans, rinsed and drained (1½ cups)

2 heirloom tomatoes, cut into wedges

4 whole pickled pepperoncini peppers

4 slices whole grain Italian bread, toasted

INSTRUCTIONS

Preheat oven to 425°F. Cut the top ¼ inch off the garlic bulb so the clove tops are exposed. Wrap bulb in foil. Roast for 40 to 50 minutes or until very soft. Let cool. Squeeze garlic from papery skin into a bowl and mash.

Meanwhile, line two baking sheets with parchment paper. Arrange artichoke hearts cut sides down on one baking sheet. In a bowl toss together radishes, kohlrabi, 1 tablespoon of the vinegar, salt, and black pepper; spread on the second baking sheet. Transfer baking sheets to oven and roast 25 minutes or until golden. Let cool to room temperature.

Meanwhile, in a medium saucepan bring broth to boiling. Add farro; reduce heat. Cover and simmer 15 minutes or until liquid is absorbed and farro is tender. Drain, if necessary. Let cool to room temperature.

To make vinaigrette, finely chop a third of the basil. Place in a small bowl. Add the remaining ½ cup balsamic vinegar; the remaining 1 clove garlic, minced; Dijon mustard, and freshly ground black pepper, to taste. Whisk to combine.

Chop the remaining basil. On a platter or in 4 shallow bowls arrange farro, artichokes, radishes, kohlrabi, beans, tomatoes, and pepperoncini peppers. Top with the chopped basil. Drizzle with basil balsamic vinaigrette. Smear toasted bread with roasted garlic; serve with platter.

Quick and Easy Grilled Veggie Brats

INGREDIENTS

1 1½-lb. daikon radish, about 12×2 inches, or 6 medium parsnips, peeled

1½ cups beer or low-sodium vegetable broth

½ cup apple cider vinegar

1 teaspoon liquid smoke

1 teaspoon dried marjoram

1 teaspoon crushed red pepper

½ teaspoon ground white pepper

⅛ teaspoon ground cloves

2½ teaspoon caraway seeds

2 sweet onions, thinly sliced

3 cloves garlic, minced

6 whole grain hot dog buns, warmed or grilled

1 cup quartered grape tomatoes

1 tablespoon coarse ground mustard

INSTRUCTIONS

Cut and trim daikon to yield six "brats" about 6×1 inches. Place daikon brats in a large saucepan; add water to cover. Bring to boiling; reduce heat. Cover and cook 9 to 13 minutes or until tender. Drain well.

Place daikon brats in a large resealable plastic bag set in a shallow dish. For marinade, in a bowl whisk together 1¼ cups of the beer, the next six ingredients (through cloves), and 2 teaspoons of the caraway seeds. Add to bag with brats; add enough water to cover. Seal bag. Chill 4 to 24 hours, turning occasionally. Drain and discard marinade.

Grill brats, covered, over medium-high 7 to 10 minutes or until grill marks appear, turning occasionally.

In a large skillet cook onions and garlic, covered, over medium 8 to 12 minutes or until tender, stirring occasionally and gradually adding remaining ¼ cup beer as needed to prevent sticking. Stir in the remaining ½ teaspoon caraway seeds.

Serve brats in buns topped with sautéed onion mixture, the tomatoes, and mustard.

Classic Mango Smoothie Bowl

INGREDIENTS

4 bananas, sliced and frozen

8 oz. orange juice (1 cup)

10 oz. frozen mango (2 cups)

1 teaspoon ground turmeric

9 oz. fresh or thawed frozen blueberries (2 cups)

2 kiwis, peeled and sliced

1 cup rolled oats

1⅓ tablespoons chia seeds

INSTRUCTIONS

In a high-powered blender (or food processor), combine orange juice, frozen bananas, frozen mango, and turmeric. Process until smooth. Pour into bowls.

Fill each bowl with blueberries, kiwi, oats, and chia seeds.

Rhubarb and Pear Tart

INGREDIENTS

1 cup cornmeal

½ cup rolled oats

2 tablespoons whole almonds

⅛ teaspoon sea salt

2 tablespoons almond butter

5 tablespoons pure maple syrup

¼ cup unsweetened, unflavored plant milk

¼ cup orange juice

1 tablespoon cornstarch

12 oz. red rhubarb, chopped into ½-inch pieces

1 pear, cored and chopped into ¼-inch pieces (1½ cups)

2 teaspoons grated fresh ginger

INSTRUCTIONS

Preheat oven to 375°F. Line the removable bottom of a 9-inch tart pan with parchment paper.

For crust, in a food processor combine cornmeal, oats, almonds, and salt. Process until almonds are ground. Add almond butter and 2 tablespoons of the maple syrup. Pulse until well combined. With processor running, slowly add milk through feed tube until mixture starts to cling together and is moistened. Press mixture over bottom and up sides of the prepared pan. Bake 10 minutes.

Meanwhile, in a medium saucepan whisk together orange juice, the remaining 3 tablespoons maple syrup, and the cornstarch. Add rhubarb, pear, and ginger. Cook and stir over medium 3 to 4 minutes or just until mixture begins to thicken.

Pour fruit mixture into partially baked crust. Bake 45 to 50 minutes or until fruit is soft and filling is thickened. Cool completely before serving.

CHAPTER V

DIETARY GUIDELINES FOR PREVENTING GALLSTONES

To reduce the risk of gallstones and promote overall gallbladder health, adhering to specific dietary guidelines is crucial. Here are some practical recommendations:

- Avoid High Energy Intake: Steer clear of high-calorie foods, especially those laden with refined sugars and unhealthy fats. These can lead to weight gain and increased risk of gallstone formation.

- Increase Fiber Intake: Aim to enrich your diet with fiber-rich foods. Incorporate plenty of fruits, vegetables, legumes, nuts, seeds, and whole grains. Fiber aids in digestion and helps maintain a healthy gallbladder.

- Opt for Healthy Fats: Choose monounsaturated fats such as those found in olive oil and avocados. These fats are less likely to contribute to gallstone formation compared to saturated and trans fats.

- Consume Omega-3 Fatty Acids: Include sources of omega-3 fatty acids, such as fatty fish, which have anti-inflammatory properties that may benefit gallbladder health.

- Moderate Alcohol Consumption: If you drink alcohol, do so in moderation. There is evidence suggesting that moderate alcohol intake may help protect against gallstones.

- Supplement Vitamin C: Consider vitamin C supplements if necessary, as vitamin C is linked to a reduced risk of gallstone formation.